The
Little
Blue
Book of
Fitness
and
Health

The
Little
Blue
Book of
Fitness
and
Health

393 Common-sense Tips to Help You
Achieve Optimum Physical, Mental, and
Spiritual Health

Gary Savage, Tony Jarvis, and Sara J. Henry

Rutledge Hill Press®
Nashville, Tennessee

Published in Nashville, Tennessee, by Rutledge Hill Press®, 211 Seventh Avenue North, Nashville, Tennessee 37219.

Distributed in Canada by H. B. Fenn & Company, Ltd., 34 Nixon Road, Bolton, Ontario L7E 1W2.

Distributed in Australia by The Five Mile Press Pty., Ltd., 22 Summit Road, Noble Park, Victoria 3174.

Distributed in New Zealand by Southern Publishers Group, 22 Burleigh Street, Grafton, Auckland.

Distributed in the United Kingdom by Verulam Publishing, Ltd., 152a Park Street Lane, Park Street, St. Albans, Hertfordshire AL2 2AU.

Typography by Compass Communications, Inc., Nashville, Tennessee
Cover design by Tim Holland
Page design by Bateman Design

Library of Congress Cataloging-in-Publication Data

The little blue book of fitness and health.
    p.   cm.
    ISBN 1-55853-674-4
    1. Health. 2. Physical fitness. 3. Nutrition. 4. Exercise.
RA776.L775   1998
613.7—dc21   98-8452
                                            CIP

Printed in the United States of America

2 3 4 5 6 7 8 9—02 01 00 99

To my family—who has always been there, through thick and thin. Thanks, I love you all.

—Gary

To my family and close friends who have made my life complete. Without all of you, I could not be half as happy as I am today.

—Tony

To Mom, who looked the other way when I rode my ten-speed all over Tennessee, and Dad, who bought me my first racing bike and drove me to bike races.

—Sara

Acknowledgments

First, we'd like to thank our publisher, Larry Stone, for all his help.

Gary offers special thanks to his parents, Gary and Sandra Savage, for always staying by his side, and Dylan Wolff, Rae Silva, Brian Faucher, Lisa Robinson, Patrick Burke, Chris Pratt, Andy Raichle, Donald Sylvestre, Dana Hanley, Jimmy Ciampi, and Laura Collins Downing for their continued friendship. Tony thanks Dr. Samuel Headley for guiding him through two very difficult years of graduate school and being a man of dignity and class; Pete Hughes for showing him the value of both intensity and compassion; and his father, Stan, for always having the right answers and giving continual guidance. Sara thanks the late Charlie Decker for pushing her to be a better writer than she ever thought she could be.

We'd also like to thank Trigg Wilkes, president of Florida YMCA Northeast, and Wendy Zinn, senior program director of Boston's Central YMCA.

Finally, we'd like to recognize and thank the staff and volunteers of Esprit De Corps and Hospice Northeast of Florida for their hard work, dedication, and friendship. You are all a special group of individuals. May God bless you as you have blessed thousands in their final hours of need.

Introduction

Many of us want to get fit. We know the benefits—the increased energy, slimmer physique, taut muscles, and stronger heart and lungs. But our lives are busy, and often we're so fatigued from daily life that we just can't find the energy to get started. Some of us might be halfway there, but need a bit of help to "get over the hump," while others are finding their daily workout routine boring and difficult to stick to.

The first thing to do is to start thinking of your fitness and health as being just as important as paying the bills, getting to work, or going to the grocery store. The second is to realize that physical, mental, and spiritual health come not from one giant step, but lots of little ones.

This book provides the guidance you need to help you start taking those little steps and to continue making them as you make fitness and health integral parts of your daily life. Its easy-to-follow tips and friendly advice will benefit anyone who wants to improve how he or she feels—from the "couch potato" just beginning to exercise, to the perpetual dieter needing an improved eating plan, to the hard-core athlete feeling a bit stale or burned out.

Pick up the book, and enjoy. We wish you a long and healthy life.

—Gary, Tony, and Sara

1.

People who exercise regularly have 36 percent lower health-care costs and 54 percent shorter hospital stays.

2.

Consult a physician before beginning any diet or exercise program.

3.

The average American diet lasts three days. Instead of dieting, make one small healthy change at a time.

4.

Get up early tomorrow and
watch the sun rise.

5.

Start slowly. Many people throw
themselves too vigorously into
an exercise program and become
hurt or discouraged.

6.

A walk around your neighborhood
after work tones your muscles,
heart, and lungs, and burns fat.

7.

Sign a written exercise contract with a friend.

8.

Have a scoop of sherbet topped with graham crackers or fruit for dessert.

9.

Experiment with healthy substitutes for your favorite foods such as mustard and salsa rather than mayonnaise, and ground turkey instead of hamburger.

10.

Rome wasn't built in a day. Neither will you create a healthy, fit body in a day or even a few weeks.

11.

Don't worry if your weight creeps up when you first start to exercise— muscle is heavier than fat. Instead of watching the scales, notice how your clothes fit.

12.

Dancing is great exercise.

13.

Need a quick snack? Grab a bagel or even a baked potato. Both steadily supply energy in the form of starches and are easy to carry on the go.

14.

Walk, don't drive, to the corner store for light shopping. At work, park a few blocks away or at the farthest end of the lot and walk.

15.

Drink a glass of water before each meal.

16.

You'll feel better and work more efficiently on twenty minutes of moderate exercise a day.

17.

A good workout program mixes aerobic exercise, such as running or swimming, with weight training. Lift weights one day and do an aerobic exercise the next.

18.

High-fiber, whole-grain cereal with low-fat milk and fruit is a healthy and delicious breakfast.

19.

Stretch, stretch, stretch. Flexible muscles are stronger and less prone to injury.

20.

Make a list of five things in your life for which you're thankful.

21.

To lure yourself into exercise, plan a reward at the end of the first three weeks—such as tickets to a sporting event or the theater.

22.

Forget the saying "No pain, no gain." You might be a bit sore after exercise sometimes, but pain is never good.

23.

The slower and farther you go, the more fat you will burn.

24.

Any exercise is better than no exercise.

25.

Find a serene place to walk or hike this weekend and give thanks for the beauty of the world around you.

26.

If a diet program or muscle-building supplement looks too good to be true, it is.

27.

As a general rule, you should burn 2,000 calories in exercise per week. (Running a mile burns 100–150 calories.)

28.

Control stress with prayer, a good book, meditation, and exercise.

29.

A potato can be a hearty and healthy meal—just avoid the butter and sour cream. Pile on vegetables, low-fat cheese, or salsa instead.

30.

There's no magic formula to weight loss. If you burn more calories than you take in, you lose weight. If you take in more calories than you burn off, you gain weight.

31.

Weight training strengthens ligaments, tendons, bones, connective tissue, and muscles.

32.

For each pound of muscle you gain from exercise, you can afford to burn off an extra 50 to 100 calories a day.

33.

The simplest way to start a running program is to walk two minutes, run two, and so on.

34.

Kiwi, papaya, cantaloupe, strawberry, mango, orange, and tangerine are all packed with calcium, folic acid, iron, protein, and vitamins.

35.

Try vegetable burgers with a few spices, catsup, and a hamburger roll for a great new taste sensation. Turkey burgers are good, too.

36.

Stretching, walking, or jogging slowly prior to exercise increases body and muscle temperature and helps decrease injuries.

37.

Adequate cool-down will decrease lactic acid, allow your heart and lungs to return to normal levels, and enhance recovery.

38.

You're never too old or out of shape to start building a healthy life.

39.

Some nutritionists believe butter is healthier than margarine because it doesn't have hydrogenated fats. All agree, however, that less is better.

40.

Enjoy your time in the pool—any movement in water burns one-third more calories than the same movement in air.

41.

Gallon water containers make convenient adjustable weights. (Just add or pour out water.)

42.

Swimming builds strength and keeps the heart and lungs healthy.

43.

Don't throw out your old clothing or furniture. Donate them to a church, Goodwill, or the Salvation Army.

44.

Substitute applesauce for shortening when baking.

45.

Allow yourself an occasional treat: Walk or bike to the store for a candy bar or a cookie.

46.

Find an exercise facility that's convenient to work or home and uncrowded at the times you want to work out. When apartment searching, check out exercise facilities.

47.

Expect some soreness when you begin an exercise program. This is part of the breakdown/build-up process that ultimately strengthens the body.

48.

It takes six weeks to form a habit.

49.

For a delicious and healthy brick-oven style pizza, buy a pizza stone, a "breathable" round ceramic stone. Make your own dough, or buy it premade at the grocery store. Add low-fat cheese, green pepper, mushrooms, and onions.

50.

Positive thinking is the key to a healthy, happy life.

51.

If you love to run but want a softer workout, take up aqua jogging—running in pools. Ask about this at your Y or health club.

52.

Pack a lunch that includes carrot sticks and an apple.

53.

Spot reducing doesn't work. Exercising a specific area tones muscles in that area, but it won't get rid of fat exclusively in one spot.

54.

When starting weight training, choose a weight that you can readily lift ten times. Add weight when you get to where you can finish your sets with relative ease.

55.

Cabbage is packed with vitamin C, potassium, folic acid, and fiber. Make a tasty coleslaw with shredded carrots and onions, mustard, and a smidgen of low-fat mayonnaise or dressing.

56.

Servings in restaurants are usually about twice as much food as you need. Divide your meal in half, and ask for a doggie bag.

57.

Be prepared for setbacks—days when you can't work out because of illness or family or work demands. Just get back into your routine as soon as possible.

58.

Squeeze half a lemon into a glass of water and add a spoonful of sugar and ice for a peppy drink. Delicious!

59.

A good basic diet is 60 to 65 percent carbohydrate, 15 percent protein, and 20 to 25 percent fat.

60.

Volunteer at your local YMCA or YWCA.

61.

Most exercise experts recommend working out at a target heart-rate zone of 70 to 80 percent of your maximum, which is roughly 220 minus your age.

62.

Keep track of your heart rate during exercise with a lightweight heart-rate monitor, available at sporting-goods stores.

63.

Drink one cup of water for every thirty minutes of exercise.

64.

A handful of dried fruits and nuts makes a quick, energy-boosting snack. Be careful not to overindulge, however, because they're high in calories.

65.

A water-exercise class can be perfect for people with arthritis or recovering from an injury, because water lets you move without stressing your body.

66.

Clean and slice carrots and celery, and put them into a plastic container in the fridge so they'll be ready for a quick snack.

67.

A good rule of thumb while training to burn fat is to maintain a pace that lets you talk.

68.

Eating too little can *slow* weight loss and hurt your health. When you drastically cut calories, your body thinks it's starving, and your metabolism slows.

69.

Create main dishes that feature pasta, rice, beans, or vegetables. Mix those foods with small amounts of lean meat, poultry, or fish.

70.

Vegetables such as peas, corn, and potatoes are nutritious—but if you're keeping track of food groups, remember that they count as carbohydrates.

71.

Aerobic exercise lowers your risk of heart disease and cancer.

72.

If you fall asleep within minutes of hitting the pillow, you're likely sleep-deprived. Most of us need eight to nine hours of sleep a night.

73.

To lose weight and keep it off, limit your weight loss to no more than one or two pounds a week.

74.

Make taking care of your body and health a top priority.

75.

Using a vegetable steamer is a delicious way to prepare vegetables—and it retains many of the vegetables' nutrients as well.

76.

As you get stronger and fitter, you'll need more of a workout—either longer or more intense—to keep getting fitter.

77.

You're never too old to lift weights. Nursing home residents, even those in wheelchairs, flourish in weight-training programs.

78.

Bike to work once a month.

79.

Believe it or not, with a regular exercise program you'll find yourself craving healthier foods. For some people, exercise even suppresses the appetite.

80.

To enliven a pool workout, use "toys" such as a pull-buoy or flutter board.

81.

Always wear your seat belt.

82.

Walking is one of the greatest exercises. Walk with your whole body—torso, hips, and legs moving smoothly and easily together, with a rolling heel-toe motion.

83.

Realize that your body gets "comfortable" at a certain weight and might be stubborn about changes. Eventually it will adjust and get used to a new set point.

84.

When joining a fitness club, get a friend to sign up, too. There's often a discount, and it's easier to stick to a routine if you have a partner.

85.

Pick a reasonable long-term goal, such as a 5K fun run six months from now.

86.

To improve your swimming stroke, sign up for an adult swim camp, such as Terry Laughlin's Total Immersion camps (800-609-SWIM).

87.

Measure all your serving sizes. You might find that you're eating two servings of cereal for breakfast and that your evening bowl of frozen yogurt is really three servings.

88.

Exercise can help relieve depression and improve self-esteem.

89.

Exercises that use the largest muscle groups—the chest, butt, and upper-leg muscles—burn the most calories. Get your Y or health-club expert to show you how.

90.

Sign up to be a Big Brother or Big Sister, or a foster parent.

91.

Trim your inner thighs with a low-intensity, long-term workout such as bicycling or running.

92.

Crash or fad diets might lead to a short-term weight loss, but almost inevitably the pounds pile back on. To lose weight permanently, exercise daily and eat more healthily.

93.

If you tend to overeat in the winter, you might need more bright lights. Many of us get wintertime blues from lack of sunshine.

94.

Make exercise a lifelong habit.

95.

Apple juice is loaded with sugar and low in nutrients. Limit it, or mix it half and half with water.

96.

Read nutrition labels. The most important information is serving size, fat, and calories. Your doctor can recommend appropriate daily calorie and fat levels, and you can then monitor your intake.

97.

"Practice moderation in all things" is a good rule.

98.

Write a mission statement for your health and fitness plans, just as you would for a big project at work.

99.

Approximately five servings a day of fruits and vegetables are recommended to stay healthy and help fend off cancer.

100.

The average person needs only one four-ounce serving of protein a day, which equates to a piece of meat about the size of a deck of cards.

101.

There is no cholesterol in grains, nuts, fruits, or vegetables—it's found only in animal products.

102.

When lifting weights for strength or power, lift between 70 and 80 percent of your maximum, with sets of six or fewer repetitions and several minutes' rest between sets.

103.

For muscle endurance, do more than twelve repetitions with lighter weights.

104.

When using free weights, ask someone to "spot" or supervise you.

105.

Two glasses of milk, a serving of yogurt, and a serving of cheese provide a healthy daily dose of calcium. Another good source is fortified juices.

106.

Try circuit training—rotating to different workout equipment with little rest in between—to beef up your workout and add variety. For best results, rest no more than sixty seconds in between.

107.

A healthier body leads to a
healthier mind.

108.

Broccoli, cabbage, green peppers,
strawberries, potatoes, and citrus
fruits are superb sources of vitamin C
and antioxidants.

109.

Get a computer program called
LifeForm (800-607-7637 or
www.lifeform.com). This dazzling
program tracks and analyzes your
daily diet, workouts, pulse rate,
and more.

110.

Regular variation in training is a must to stimulate muscle growth and improvement—and to prevent boredom!

111.

Drink seven or eight glasses of water a day—even more fluids if exercising.

112.

To prevent low-back pain, work on building your lower-back muscles, as well as stretching hip flexors and quadriceps.

113.

Salmon, sardines, herring, mackerel, cod, and haddock are packed with protein—and a type of healthy fat with lots of heart-healthy benefits.

114.

Keep plenty of watermelon on hand during the summer months.

115.

Use a waterproof sunscreen.

116.

Avoid eating late in the evening so that your body will have time to burn off calories before you go to sleep.

117.

Gains come systematically and over time.

118.

A candy bar can supply a quick (but brief) energy boost. To avoid roller-coaster energy levels, eat more complex carbohydrates such as potatoes, pasta, grain, and vegetables.

119.

For inexpensive, nutritious, and low-fat protein, try beans, split peas, and lentils. You can buy them cooked or easily prepare the dried variety.

120.

Hard candy contains less fat and fewer calories than chocolate bars, potato chips, or other snacks.

121.

Wash your fruits and vegetables thoroughly before eating them.

122.

Everyone is different. Don't expect to be able to do what your neighbor or the guy across the gym is doing.

123.

Keep an exercise log in a notebook— jot down your workout and how you felt. This can help you to get motivated, to recognize workout and fatigue patterns, and to avoid injury.

124.

Try out a new activity this year, such as cross-country skiing, kayaking, yoga, or in-line skating.

125.

Avoid the temptation to take a long layoff from working out because of work or vacation. Squeeze in a workout, no matter how short.

126.

Create your own sports drink by mixing fruit juice half and half with water.

127.

Take along a pair of tennis shoes and a swimsuit when traveling. Even a brief swim can help. If there's no pool, take a half-hour walk, outdoors or in.

128.

Choose baked or grilled foods over fried.

129.

Go easy on the doughnuts: They're loaded with artery-clogging fat.

130.

For resistance training when out of town, use rubberized workout bands or portable weights that you fill up with water.

131.

Take a tennis or racquetball lesson.

132.

When you wake up in the morning, repeat a positive thought to yourself. Say, "I'm going to have a good day today," or "I'm proud of how I've been working out."

133.

Hang a framed sign outlining your fitness goals in your home or office.

134.

Weight training will increase your strength and give you more energy for day-to-day tasks.

135.

When at a fitness club, ask a trainer to demonstrate all the equipment.

136.

Train year-round—there's no such thing as an off-season! The different seasons offer a multitude of wonderful cross-training activities.

137.

Sign up for a CPR course.

138.

Great, super low-calorie vegetables include green beans, spinach, broccoli, cauliflower, zucchini, carrots, celery, and cabbage. Indulge!

139.

Steer clear of supplements that promise to enhance muscle development.

140.

Make salad an important part of your meal plan. Instead of iceberg or head lettuce, which has few nutrients, choose a darker variety such as romaine or leaf lettuce.

141.

Salsa is a delicious fat-free dip or topping.

142.

Don't work out when ill or seriously injured. Your body needs time and energy to heal and recover.

143.

Look at serving sizes on nutrition labels. You might think that a breakfast muffin is a great low-calorie choice, but that's only if you eat half the muffin.

144.

Before traveling, ask your gym if there are any fitness centers at your destination with reciprocal agreements.

145.

Train your mind as well as your body:
Plan an activity for the coming
months that stretches your mind.
Sign up for a class or read some
thought-provoking books.

146.

Read articles about health and fitness,
but be wary of "fads" and tips based
on a single study.

147.

Help someone less fortunate than you.

148.

Working out every day might be too much. Give your body some time off.

149.

Choose pretzels over potato chips.

150.

Create opportunities for exercise.

151.

Water is nature's soft drink.

152.

Try some isometric exercises: By pressing against immovable objects or simply contracting your muscles, you can get a workout almost anywhere without equipment.

153.

Choose lunch delis that offer foods such as chicken, turkey, salads, fruits, and vegetables.

154.

Proper form is important whether you're lifting weights, running, or swimming—it saves energy, is more efficient, and helps prevent injury.

155.

Put up a basketball hoop in your driveway and organize neighborhood games.

156.

While at the movies, ask for "air-popped" popcorn without added butter. Better yet, buy pretzels or Twizzlers.

157.

Try a slideboard: It gives a great leg workout with little or no stress on the joints, and it will improve your posture and balance.

158.

Schedule your workout to fit your lifestyle. A 6:00 A.M. workout might wake you up and invigorate you—or one after work can dissipate your job stress.

159.

Enjoy pasta with red sauce. Avoid or limit Alfredo, cream, and buttery sauces. Experiment with making your own sauces from wine and herbs.

160.

Learn the Heimlich maneuver.

161.

Remove turkey and chicken skin—it's loaded with fat. When possible, choose white meat over red meat.

162.

Ask a co-worker to jog with you at lunch, or a neighbor to walk with you after work. It can be a great motivator.

163.

Eat a variety of foods every day.

164.

Take the time to thank the maintenance crew at your fitness club. Let them know what a great job they do.

165.

Avoid exercising on either a full or an empty stomach.

166.

To hydrate for a run or long bike ride, drink several glasses of water at least an hour before you start.

167.

Before strength training, do six to ten minutes of aerobic exercise to get your muscles warmed up and ready.

168.

Encourage children to join the Boy Scouts and Girl Scouts of America. Volunteer to help their leaders.

169.

Take the stairs whenever possible.

170.

Buy a quality mattress and bedding materials. We spend a third of our life sleeping, and better rest will help with exercise recovery.

171.

Bananas might be nature's most perfect food.

172.

Protein alone doesn't build muscle; exercise plus healthy food choices do.

173.

It should take twice as long to lower a weight than to raise it. Count *one-thousand, two-thousand,* etc., to keep track.

174.

Instead of using a commercial diet plan that sells prepacked meals, make intelligent food choices and fix your own healthy meals.

175.

Your best workout partner might be your spouse or significant other.

176.

Try tofu (soybean curd) in casseroles or stews. It's an excellent low-fat protein source.

177.

Music can be a great motivator: Consider using a headset radio or tape player when exercising indoors. Make your own workout tape of songs that energize you.

178.

Visit an elderly person in a nursing home.

179.

Switch to nonfat and low-fat dairy products—such as cottage cheese and frozen yogurt. They taste noticeably different at first but your palate will soon adjust.

180.

A "low-fat" label doesn't mean nonfattening! Many companies compensate for the change in taste by adding sugar.

181.

Get a massage.
It's wonderfully relaxing
and helps your
muscles recover.

182.

Your muscles need a full forty-eight hours to recover and rebuild after a weight workout, and sometimes more.

183.

Pray every day.

184.

Participate in a local road race or walk-a-thon that raises money for charity. It's great fun and involves you in the community.

185.

To help lower your blood pressure, eat more fruits, grains, dairy products, and vegetables.

186.

When dining out, ask for salad dressing on the side instead of pouring the dressing on your salad. Dip your fork into it before each bite.

187.

A pet can be a great companion and wonderful company on runs and walks.

188.

Peanut butter and nuts are good
protein sources with no cholesterol.
But they're high in calories,
so take it easy.

189.

Pick up a copy of Tom Anderson's
Stretching (800-333-1307, or look in
your bookstore). Stretch lightly
before a workout and more
extensively afterward.

190.

Some insurance companies offer
lower rates for runners. Just ask.

191.

Moderate wine drinking (no more than one glass a day) may have some health benefits.

192.

Subscribe to a few health magazines. They offer useful information and help motivate you.

193.

Consider using egg substitutes or egg whites instead of whole eggs. Some nutritionists recommend no more than three to four egg yolks per week.

194.

Make a great summer refresher by blending ice and fruits.

195.

Plan for the holidays. If your fitness center or gym will be closed, schedule a day off or plan for an outside exercise.

196.

When you increase the weight you're lifting, increase by no more than 5 percent at a time.

197.

Nothing beats waking to the aroma of freshly baked bread. Set a bread maker to have a loaf ready in the morning.

198.

Try a scoop of frozen yogurt topped with lots of fresh fruit.

199.

The best gauge for checking your body fat is seeing how you look in the mirror and how you fit into your clothes.

200.

Don't just watch those aerobic programs on television—follow along!

201.

Eat your toast or bagel plain or with jam or jelly. Ditch the cream cheese, butter, and margarine.

202.

Steamed rice, vegetables, and skinless chicken with spices make a delicious low-fat meal. Brown rice is the best choice.

203.

Take the time to compliment others
on a good workout.

204.

When using exercise facilities,
use a towel to clean up your sweat at
each station, and return equipment
where it goes.

205.

Never ignore pain around the joints.
If it becomes severe or persists, head
for your doctor's office.

206.

A fitness club is a great place to meet new people, form friendships, and even make business contacts.

207.

Sign up for a club or team—softball, volleyball, rowing, or any other sport that interests you.

208.

An outdoor grill is a healthy way to prepare meats. Grilled vegetables are delicious, too.

209.

Don't let the weather dictate your exercise schedule. Substitute an indoor workout, or dress for the weather and go for it!

210.

Get a complete physical exam at least once a year.

211.

Enjoy a healthy snack such as fruit or rice cakes between meals. This gives you energy, reduces your appetite, and increases your metabolism.

212.

For weight workouts, it's important to keep records that include the date, weight lifted, number of repetitions, and time spent working out.

213.

Choose restaurants that offer healthy meals. Look for symbols on menus that indicate dishes lower in fat, cholesterol, and calories.

214.

Send a thank-you card to someone who has helped you in your life.

215.

To figure the approximate number of calories you burn per mile of walking or light jogging, multiply your weight in pounds by .77.

216.

Instead of registering for china for your wedding, register for sporting equipment at L. L. Bean, Eddie Bauer, Eastern Mountains Sports, and other sports outfitters.

217.

Exercise slows the aging process.

218.

Breathe out when you lift a weight,
and inhale when you lower it.

219.

Saturated fat is harmful. Consume no
more than ten grams a day.

220.

Volunteer at a summer camp
for children.

221.

When making a plane reservation, request a low-fat or healthy meal. Most airlines will accommodate you at no additional cost.

222.

Use skim milk or nonfat creamer in your coffee.

223.

Listening to soothing music relieves stress.

224.

Many "gym rats" overdevelop front muscles—the ones they see in the mirror—and neglect the back. Keep muscle development balanced.

225.

It's okay to say no when someone offers you a cookie, candy, pastry, or doughnut.

226.

Start an enduring family tradition now: Take family walks together.

227.

Alternate muscle groups during a workout so your muscles can recover between exercises.

228.

Substitute an orange for your evening snack of chips or nuts.

229.

Cook healthy while adding flavor. Use spices, garlic, and herbs.

230.

Be a role model for your children and others when it comes to exercise and nutrition.

231.

Think about what is most important in your life.

232.

If your exercise partner is on vacation, busy, or sick, work out alone. Don't miss your workout because others do.

233.

When golfing, walk whenever possible. You'll see more of the beautiful scenery on the course.

234.

The holiday season doesn't mean it's time to overindulge and stop exercising.

235.

While at the beach, take a long walk or run.

236.

Ask people who are healthy and fit how they do it.

237.

Get a wooden banana hanger and keep it full.

238.

Participate in contests at your fitness club.

239.

Wear your favorite college or professional team's logo when you exercise. This is a great way to meet people.

240.

Before you eat pizza, pat the top with paper napkins to remove excess oil, and ask for less cheese and extra sauce when ordering.

241.

If friends or family are trying to change eating habits or begin an exercise program, encourage them. They'll be pleased.

242.

Avoid cooking with coconut oil or lard. The healthiest oils are olive, canola, and safflower.

243.

Try Healthy Choice pizza—it's great French bread pizza with only one gram of fat.

244.

Make a list of twenty-five things you want to do in your lifetime. Start planning now to do at least one a year.

245.

Low-fat cereals such as Wheat Chex make a great snack. Heat them with a little olive oil and garlic, and add raisins and dried fruit. (Most cereals have recipes on the box.)

246.

Go hiking in a national or state park.

247.

Be sure your running shoes fit well. Check out the *Runners World* home page at www.runnersworld.com to select the right shoe for you.

248.

Make it a household rule:
one hour of television for each hour
of study or exercise.

249.

Jell-O with fruit is a great dessert.

250.

For your next vacation, try an
organized bike tour: It's an unbeatable
way to visit new areas. Try Vermont
Bicycle Tours (800-BIKE-TOUR or
www.vbt.com).

251.

Impress your date with a healthy home-cooked meal.

252.

Take fruit with you to your fitness club or to the park where you run or bike. It makes for a tasty treat when you're finished.

253.

Alternate high, medium, and light days in your weight workouts—in addition to taking days off in between.

254.

Granola might taste great, but it can be loaded with fat and calories. Check the label.

255.

Stash an exercise bar such as PowerBar in your fanny pack, gym bag, or bike bag. Running out of fuel is no fun and may result in injury.

256.

Avoid exercising outdoors in extreme temperatures. It's not worth the health risks.

257.

Drink a carbohydrate-electrolyte beverage such as Gatorlode during moderate to high-intensity aerobic exercise that lasts more than ninety minutes.

258.

For any aerobic exercise less than ninety minutes, water is the best choice.

259.

At restaurants, ask for your vegetables without butter. Avoid cream sauces and fried foods.

260.

Eat pasta with a vegetarian tomato-based sauce the night before a road race.

261.

Sign up for an indoor cycling, or "spinning," class.

262.

Ask a certified fitness instructor to design an exercise routine for you.

263.

Buy (and use) healthy cookbooks.

264.

Add sprouts to your sandwiches.

265.

Stretch for at least ten minutes before going to bed. This will help release stress and induce a good night's sleep.

266.

When performing weight-training exercises that stress the lower back, use a weight-lifting belt to prevent injuries to your middle torso area and spine.

267.

Start a "healthy dinner club" with half a dozen friends. Meet once a week and swap cooking duties.

268.

Many employers offer "fitness time"—if yours doesn't, ask. Healthy employees are efficient employees.

269.

When invited to a formal event, request a vegetarian meal with your RSVP.

270.

While exercising, wear comfortable and functional clothing. Modern wicking fibers allow sweat to evaporate and keep you from getting soggy.

271.

Enjoy a steam bath or sauna to relax your muscles and mind.

272.

Women who find bicycling more painful than enjoyable might want to try just-for-women products by Terry Precision Bicycles (800-289-8379).

273.

Apricots are a good source of fiber and loaded with vitamin A—and each has only seventeen calories.

274.

Be romantic at breakfast—squeeze orange juice for your partner and serve it in bed.

275.

Always keep grapes in your refrigerator, ready to eat.

276.

Exercise reduces stress-related chemicals in your body and pumps out feel-good endorphins.

277.

Milk is an excellent source of vitamin D and calcium, nutrients that keep bones healthy. Salmon and tuna also pack a vitamin D punch.

278.

Tape-measure your waist, chest, and arms every four to six weeks.

279.

For a quick indoor warm-up, try running in place for two to three minutes.

280.

Sit-ups and push-ups are good exercises—if you do them correctly. Don't lunge, and keep your back straight.

281.

Subscribe to *Consumer Reports*. Start here when purchasing new exercise equipment, bikes, in-line skates, etc.

282.

Shrimp, crab, and lobster are great— as long as you don't dip them in butter. Try them in tomato sauce on pasta.

283.

Make it a point to attend church, even on the road.

284.

A fresh melon at breakfast looks great on the table and on your body.

285.

Sign up for one of L. L. Bean's
Outdoor Discovery Schools
(800-341-4341, extension 6666).

286.

Start your meal with salad instead
of bread.

287.

Practice soothing breathing when
you find yourself tensing up.
Count backward slowly from ten, and
picture the tension leaving your body.

288.

Pick up some books on tape (available at your local library) to listen to while exercising indoors.

289.

Keep small hand weights stashed under your sofa to use while watching TV.

290.

People who work out have a more positive self-image, stronger self-esteem, and an improved sense of well-being.

291.

Never quit dreaming.
You must first dream
something before you
can accomplish it.

292.

Oatmeal is a filling, nutritious breakfast. Add sliced bananas or raisins.

293.

Buy an ocean kayak and enjoy the sights. Explore a harbor, river, or lake at dawn or dusk.

294.

Treat yourself to fresh peaches, strawberries, and plums.

295.

Take an Outward Bound trip: It'll change your life. (Call 800-243-8520.)

296.

When tailgating at a sporting event, bring a picnic basket filled with fruits and vegetables. Grill boneless, skinless chicken and vegetables.

297.

If someone is using the exercise machine you want, move on to the next one and come back later. Keep moving.

298.

Encourage your children to participate in team sports. Besides providing exercise, these teach the importance of being a team player.

299.

Fig bars are great energy-boosting, fiber-filled snacks.

300.

Vacation in a place like Maine or Oregon, where you can enjoy the ocean, mountains, rivers, and lakes— all in the same week.

301.

Put those too-snug clothes in plain sight as fitness incentives.

302.

Always ask for help—physical, mental, or spiritual—when you need it.

303.

Use your car or a bicycle to map mileage for your walking, running, or biking route.

304.

At a hotel, ask for the best place to run or walk, and for specific landmarks to avoid getting lost.

305.

Coffee can provide a lift, but limit yourself to four cups a day. Try switching to half-decaf, half-regular.

306.

Take time for God, yourself, and your family.

307.

Most football and baseball stadiums offer a lower-fat hot dog and other healthy substitutes.

308.

Plan a detailed four- to six-month exercise routine for those long, cold winter months.

309.

Buy a mountain bike and helmet— most ski areas and many parks have mountain bike trails.

310.

Join a recreational league or fitness club basketball team.

311.

Get a current copy of your local parks and recreation department's seasonal brochure of events and facilities.

312.

Attend an Easter sunrise service.

313.

Keep your exercise bag packed and ready to go for exercise after a hard day of work.

314.

Splurge on a personal trainer when beginning a new fitness routine. Team up with a friend and share the cost.

315.

Improve your flexibility with swimming, cross-country skiing, or aerobics.

316.

Before you reach for a snack, try a glass of water first.

317.

Adolescents should train for muscular endurance—doing more than twelve repetitions with lighter weights—and not for strength or power.

318.

Steer clear of buffalo wings, cheese fries, and fried potato skins. Eat cheese in moderation.

319.

Juices provide necessary fluids plus some nutrients, but they're high-calorie as well. Eating an orange or two is more beneficial than drinking orange juice.

320.

Stay motivated—never give up!

321.

Allergies to peanuts, nuts, fish, and shellfish can be severe and life-threatening. Doctors advise *not giving* these foods to children until they are at least two years old.

322.

Always find time for spiritual growth,
no matter how busy you are.

323.

Raisins are a compact energy source,
loaded with nutrients. Sprinkle them
on your breakfast cereal.

324.

Take advantage of cold weather—
try cross-country skiing, ice skating,
or snowshoeing.

325.

Think "whole body" when it comes
to health.

326.

Be aware that if you gradually gain
weight over the years, you won't lose
it all in a week (or even a month).

327.

To work out, select enjoyable
activities, places, times, equipment—
and partners.

328.

Exercise a minimum of twenty to thirty minutes, three to five times a week to keep your heart healthy. Even more is better, says the American College of Sports Medicine.

329.

If you're revamping your diet, clean out your kitchen cupboards. Ditch the chips and other unhealthy snacks.

330.

Never go grocery shopping when you're hungry!

331.

Limit soda pop—even the diet variety. Artificial sweeteners, while noncaloric, can stimulate your appetite.

332.

Surround yourself with people who share your goals and encourage you.

333.

Beware of exercise gadgets or diets advertised by celebrities: Remember, they're getting paid to promote these things.

334.

Water is all you need to drink while training with weights. Downing a sports drink or eating carbohydrates *after* a strength workout can help your muscles and body recover.

335.

Watch other people work out. You'll see new exercises to try.

336.

Reflective vests and flashing strobe lights let drivers see you when you're exercising after dark. This could save your life.

337.

By switching to skim milk, you can save 7.6 grams of fat a day—or six pounds of fat in a year.

338.

Rest is the only cure to the overtraining blues.

339.

Face traffic when running or walking on a road with no sidewalk. When biking, however, ride *with* traffic, not against it.

340.

Sign up to help an adult learn how to read.

341.

Freeze different juices in your ice-cube trays, with toothpicks as "popsicle" sticks. Your kids will love them.

342.

Help Santa lose weight.
Leave fruit and vegetables instead of cookies and brownies.

343.

One of the best ways to avoid osteoporosis—thinning of the bones that can lead to debilitating breaks—is to start a weight-training program now. Exercise helps build strong bones.

344.

It's a lot easier to put
on fat than to
take it off!

345.

Abdominal crunches help build stomach muscles. But you won't see those abs unless you also exercise aerobically and eat right.

346.

Go apple picking with your family in the fall (or berry picking in the spring and summer) and literally enjoy the fruits of your labor!

347.

Being active is the key to improving muscular strength, endurance, flexibility, and body composition.

348.

Always keep your mind open to the wide range of possible activities. Variety is the spice of life.

349.

Think fitter, faster, and stronger.

350.

If you've ever thought about running a marathon, start training today.

351.

Use good posture while walking or working. Bad alignment stresses your spine, neck, and other muscles.

352.

Buy a biking helmet and always wear it when you ride.

353.

Studies have shown that vitamin E can benefit people with heart trouble. Some doctors recommend four hundred International Units (IU) of vitamin E daily.

354.

An evening stroll around the neighborhood doesn't merit a second slice of pie for dessert.

355.

Sweet potatoes sliced into french-fry shapes and baked make a tasty, nutritious treat. Serve with turkey burgers for a great casual meal.

356.

Just because low-fat is good, don't assume that no fat is better. Fat is an essential nutrient your body needs.

357.

If you want a stepping workout and don't have stairs, use a box or stool six to twelve inches high, and do twenty minutes of continuous stepping.

358.

Chill soups and stews after cooking, and remove the solidified fat from the top. Trim the fat off meats before cooking.

359.

Organize your training into cycles of training objectives and tasks to prevent overtraining. This practice is called *periodization.*

360.

Greens such as spinach and collard greens might help avoid a serious eye problem (macular degeneration). Eat two or three helpings a week.

361.

Organize a group of friends to meet at the park and play a game of Ultimate Frisbee or volleyball.

362.

Too rushed and hungry to cook dinner? Load up a Crock-Pot in the morning and have tasty stews or soups piping hot and ready to eat at dinnertime.

363.

Losing as little as ten pounds can radically benefit overweight people with type 2 diabetes.

364.

You can help lower bad cholesterol (LDL) through healthy eating, and raise your good-cholesterol levels (HDL) through exercise.

365.

Don't confuse lots of sweat with a great workout.

366.

If you have a mole that's changed shape or color—or is asymmetrical, has an irregular border, or is bigger than a pencil eraser—get to a dermatologist without delay.

367.

Take a walking tour of historic sites.

368.

It can be tough to get all the minerals and vitamins you need. A balanced multivitamin and mineral supplement such as Centrum is good insurance.

369.

A taco salad has more fat than most large hamburgers—largely because the shell is loaded with four hundred calories and twenty grams of fat!

370.

Choose baked tortillas instead of fried ones.

371.

To improve grip strength, squeeze a tennis ball or hand grips while riding in a car or reading.

372.

Plan one day doing just what you choose—whether it's spending all day at the movies, cycling through the countryside, or browsing old book stores.

373.

Pork tenderloin and skinless turkey and chicken breasts are high in protein and low in fat.

374.

Don't lean on the rails of stair climbers—let your arms hang naturally or keep a light touch on the rails for balance. To burn more calories, take deeper steps.

375.

Think of meat as a condiment, not the centerpiece of your meal.

376.

Choose "fat-free" or "light" mayonnaise.

377.

Beware of body-fat tests, whether with calipers or by electrical impedance. There's a big margin of error, especially if the tester isn't well-trained.

378.

Doing your own landscaping and handyman duties is an excellent way to increase your activity level.

379.

Volunteer to help others at least once a month.

380.

No man is too macho to take an aerobics class.

381.

Zinc lozenges can help reduce the duration of a cold.

382.

Enroll your children in swimming lessons at an early age.

383.

Exercise, combined with
adequate rest,
can strengthen your
immune system.

384.

Do something fun with your family this weekend. Go for a walk or a bike ride or take them to a park for a picnic.

385.

Leave your badminton or volleyball net up all summer. Mark boundaries by mowing around them.

386.

A membership to the local fitness club makes a nice birthday gift. Some offer one-month or thirty-visit options.

387.

Cross-country skiing works more muscles—and does it more gently—than just about any other exercise. A good Nordic machine will do the same.

388.

Train for balance of opposing muscle groups, such as your quads and hamstrings. Any serious muscle imbalances might result in injury. Consult a fitness professional.

389.

A bagel with peanut butter is a quick and easy breakfast—a nice balance of protein and carbohydrates to start the day.

390.

When grilling, a slower fire will cook out more fat, especially with hamburgers. Also, darker ground beef has less fat than lighter ground beef.

391.

Choose comfortable and well-fitting shoes—both for daily wear and for working out. Poorly fitted shoes stress your muscles and damage your feet.

392.

Make a lifetime pledge to fitness.

393.

Take time to watch the sun set today.